Cardio Workouts For The Aging Body

Enhance Heart Health, Energize Your Body, and Embrace Vitality at Every Stage of Life

Basil U

COPYRIGHT

TABLE OF CONTENTS

ABOUT THE BOOK

As we age, maintaining physical health becomes increasingly vital. "Cardio Workouts for the Aging Body: Golden Aerobics" is a comprehensive guide designed specifically for seniors who want to embrace an active lifestyle through aerobic exercise. This book combines practical advice, scientific insights, and engaging storytelling to empower older adults to prioritize their cardiovascular health and overall well-being.

Purpose and Vision

The primary purpose of this book is to demystify cardio workouts for seniors and encourage them to integrate aerobic exercise into their daily routines. With a focus on accessibility, safety, and enjoyment, "Golden Aerobics" aims to help older adults discover the joys and benefits of staying active. It provides the tools needed to build confidence and competence in engaging in physical activity, ultimately fostering a healthier, happier life.

Importance of Cardio for Seniors

As we age, our bodies undergo various changes that can impact health and mobility. Cardiovascular diseases, reduced lung capacity, and decreased muscle strength can become more prevalent, making it crucial to prioritize heart-healthy activities. Aerobic exercise not only strengthens the heart but also improves circulation, enhances respiratory function, and boosts overall energy levels. This book explores how regular cardio workouts can combat common age-related challenges, improve mood, and promote cognitive function.

A Holistic Approach

"Golden Aerobics" takes a holistic approach to fitness, recognizing that exercise is just one component of a healthy lifestyle. The book addresses important aspects of wellness, including nutrition, hydration, and recovery. By emphasizing the interconnectedness of physical activity and overall health, readers will gain a comprehensive understanding of how to optimize their well-being.

Structure and Content

The book is structured to guide readers through their fitness journey step by step. Each chapter is packed with practical tips, tailored workouts, and inspiring stories from seniors who have successfully incorporated cardio into their lives. Topics include:

- The Benefits of Cardio: Understanding how aerobic exercise impacts heart health, mental well-being, and physical mobility.
- Getting Started Safely: Consulting healthcare providers, listening to one's body, and creating personalized fitness plans.
- Low-Impact Cardio Options: Exploring various exercises such as walking, water aerobics, and chair workouts that are gentle on joints while providing effective cardiovascular benefits.

- Golden Aerobics Routines: Tailored routines that include moderate-intensity workouts, interval training, and fun activities like dance.

- Managing Age-Related Challenges: Strategies for adapting workouts to accommodate arthritis, heart conditions, and other common health issues.

- Cognitive Function and Social Engagement: The connection between cardio workouts and brain health, highlighting the benefits of group fitness for social interaction and motivation.

- Nutrition and Recovery: Guidance on fueling the aging body, hydration tips, and the importance of rest for long-term fitness success.

- Creating Long-Term Habits: Strategies for staying motivated, tracking progress, and overcoming fitness plateaus.

- Special Populations: Customized cardio options for seniors with diabetes, respiratory conditions, and limited mobility, ensuring inclusivity and accessibility.

Inspiring Stories and Practical Tips

Throughout the book, readers will find personal anecdotes from seniors who have successfully transformed their lives through aerobic exercise. These stories serve as motivation and relatable examples, illustrating that it is never too late to start prioritizing health. Each chapter includes practical tips and sample workouts, making it easy for readers to implement what they learn.

"Cardio Workouts for the Aging Body: Golden Aerobics" is not just a fitness manual; it's a celebration of the vibrant lives that can be lived at any age. By empowering seniors to embrace physical activity, this book aims to inspire a movement toward healthier, happier aging. With its accessible language and engaging storytelling, "Golden Aerobics" encourages readers to step confidently into their fitness journey, equipped with the knowledge and tools to thrive in their golden years.

Join us in this exploration of health and wellness, and discover how cardio workouts can enhance your quality of life, fostering strength, vitality, and joy in every step.

INTRODUCTION

As we journey through life, our bodies undergo a series of changes that can sometimes feel daunting. With each passing year, we might find ourselves reminiscing about our youthful vigor and agility. However, embracing aerobic exercise during our later years can redefine this narrative, turning what could be a story of decline into one of vitality and resilience.

Cardiovascular health is paramount for seniors. Engaging in aerobic exercise—activities that increase your heart rate and improve blood circulation—offers numerous benefits, from boosting energy levels to enhancing mental clarity. As we age, our bodies need support to maintain cardiovascular health, and aerobic exercises serve as a crucial pillar in this foundation. Regular cardio workouts can lower the risk of chronic diseases, improve mobility, and even lift our spirits. This book is a guide to rediscovering joy in movement and understanding how aerobic activities can enrich our lives as we grow older.

Yet, despite these clear benefits, many older adults grapple with misconceptions and fears surrounding exercise. Common worries include the belief that cardio workouts are too strenuous or that they could lead to injury. These barriers can prevent individuals from embracing an active lifestyle, leaving them feeling isolated or disconnected from their bodies. It's essential to challenge these notions. Aerobic exercise is not just for the young and fit; it's adaptable, and there are myriad ways to incorporate it safely into our daily routines.

Let's address these fears head-on. First, it's vital to recognize that cardio can be tailored to individual capabilities. Whether you're a seasoned athlete or someone who's just starting, there's a place for you in the world of aerobic exercise. From leisurely walks in the park to invigorating water aerobics, options abound that can accommodate various fitness levels and preferences. By focusing on what our bodies can do rather than what they can't, we can shift our mindset from one of limitation to one of empowerment.

To better understand the significance of aerobic exercise for seniors, we must delve into how aging impacts the cardiovascular system. As we age, our hearts may not pump as vigorously, and our blood vessels can become stiffer, affecting overall circulation. This natural decline can be mitigated through consistent aerobic activity, which strengthens the heart muscle, enhances circulation, and increases lung capacity. Engaging in cardio workouts can effectively combat some of the adverse effects of aging, allowing us to maintain independence and mobility.

This book will not only explore the science behind aerobic exercise but also weave in stories of individuals who have embraced these workouts later in life. You'll meet Clara, who found her passion for dancing in a senior aerobics class, and Henry, who discovered the joy of cycling after retirement. Their journeys highlight that it's never too late to start, and the rewards of engaging in aerobic activities extend far beyond physical fitness.

In addition to personal anecdotes, this guide is designed to provide practical advice and resources. Each chapter will offer insights into safe practices, tailored workout options, and tips for overcoming the hurdles that often accompany starting a new exercise regime. You'll learn about low-impact alternatives that make cardio accessible, ways to stay motivated, and strategies to incorporate aerobic activities into your everyday life seamlessly.

Through this exploration, we aim to create a supportive community that fosters connection and encouragement among seniors. The power of shared experiences can be transformative, reminding us that we are not alone on this journey. As we share our successes and setbacks, we can inspire one another to stay active and engaged.

As you turn the pages of this book, remember that every step taken towards a more active lifestyle is a step towards a healthier, happier you. Aerobic exercise is not merely a means to an end; it's an invitation to embrace life fully, with all its challenges and joys. Let's embark on this journey together, rediscovering the pleasure of movement and the strength that comes from taking care of our bodies as we age.

Welcome to "Golden Aerobic" : a celebration of life, vitality, and the enduring power of cardio workouts in our later years. Let's dive in and explore how we can embrace this vibrant phase of life, one aerobic step at a time.

CHAPTER 1

BENEFITS OF CARDIO FOR THE AGING BODY

As we age, the notion of fitness may evolve, but the importance of cardiovascular health remains steadfast. Cardio workouts are often viewed through the lens of youth, but they hold remarkable benefits for older adults, enhancing not just physical well-being but also mental and emotional health. Let's explore how aerobic exercise can profoundly impact various aspects of our lives.

Heart Health: Strengthening the Heart and Improving Circulation

At the core of our cardiovascular system lies the heart, a vital organ that pumps life-sustaining blood throughout our bodies. As we age, the heart's efficiency can diminish; however, regular aerobic exercise can combat this decline. Engaging in activities like walking, swimming, or cycling strengthens the heart muscle, improving its ability to pump blood more effectively.

Take Ruth, for instance, a sprightly 72-year-old who began walking briskly every morning after her doctor emphasized the importance of heart health. Initially, she struggled with shortness of breath, but as weeks passed, her stamina grew, and she could walk longer distances without difficulty. Routine check-ups revealed improved blood pressure and cholesterol levels, validating her efforts. Ruth's story exemplifies how dedicating time to cardio can significantly enhance heart health, making everyday activities easier and more enjoyable.

Respiratory Benefits: Enhancing Lung Capacity and Breathing Efficiency

Aerobic exercise also plays a crucial role in respiratory health. With age, lung capacity may decrease, leading to reduced oxygen intake. However, consistent cardio activities can increase lung efficiency, allowing for deeper and more effective breathing. This is particularly beneficial for older adults, as improved respiratory function can enhance overall energy levels and endurance.

Consider George, who, at 68, found himself easily fatigued after minimal exertion. He joined a local tai chi class, which emphasized controlled movements and focused breathing. Over time, George noticed a remarkable difference in his ability to perform everyday tasks, like climbing stairs or carrying groceries. His increased lung capacity not only made physical activities easier but also contributed to a greater sense of well-being and vitality.

Mental Health & Mood Boost: Reducing Anxiety, Depression, and Cognitive Decline

The mental health benefits of aerobic exercise cannot be overstated. Physical activity stimulates the release of endorphins, the body's natural mood lifters. Regular cardio can significantly reduce symptoms of anxiety and depression, providing a sense of accomplishment and purpose.

Marjorie, a retired teacher, found herself feeling increasingly isolated after losing her husband. A friend encouraged her to join a community walking group. Initially hesitant, Marjorie took the plunge, and soon, the camaraderie and fresh air lifted her spirits. Not only did her mood improve, but she also noticed her cognitive function becoming sharper. Research indicates that aerobic exercise can enhance brain health, potentially lowering the risk of cognitive decline and dementia. Marjorie's journey illustrates the profound impact that social interaction and physical activity can have on mental health.

Bone Density & Joint Mobility: Reducing the Risk of Osteoporosis and Improving Joint Health

As we age, the risk of osteoporosis and joint problems increases. Cardio workouts, particularly weight-bearing exercises, can help maintain and improve bone density. Activities like dancing, walking, and even stair climbing promote bone health by putting stress on the bones, which stimulates bone growth and strength.

Harold, a 75-year-old retired engineer, faced challenges with stiffness in his knees. After consulting with his doctor, he incorporated low-impact aerobics and stretching routines into his weekly schedule. Over time, he experienced improved joint mobility and reduced discomfort. Regular cardio not only helped him maintain his independence but also enabled him to participate in activities he loved, like gardening and playing with his grandchildren.

Metabolism & Weight Management: Maintaining a Healthy Weight and Metabolic Function

Maintaining a healthy weight is crucial for overall health, especially as our metabolism naturally slows with age. Engaging in regular aerobic exercise can boost metabolic function, making it easier to manage weight. Moreover, cardio workouts help burn calories, supporting weight loss or maintenance while improving body composition.

Linda, a 69-year-old grandmother, struggled with weight gain after retirement. Determined to reclaim her health, she started attending a water aerobics class at her local community center. The buoyancy of the water made it easier on her joints while providing a vigorous workout. Over the months, Linda not only shed extra pounds but also felt more energetic and vibrant. Her success story serves as a testament to the effectiveness of cardio in weight management and overall vitality.

The Transformative Power of Cardio

In summary, the benefits of cardiovascular exercise for seniors are vast and varied. From enhancing heart health and lung capacity to boosting mental well-being and supporting bone strength, aerobic activities are a vital component of healthy aging. The stories of individuals like Ruth, George, Marjorie, Harold, and Linda remind us that it's never too late to embark on a journey toward better health.

As you consider integrating more cardio into your life, remember that the most important aspect is finding activities that you enjoy. Whether it's dancing, walking, swimming, or group classes, embracing a variety of exercises can make your fitness journey more enjoyable and sustainable.

In the following chapters, we will delve into how to get started safely, create personalized fitness plans, and explore a range of enjoyable cardio activities tailored specifically for the aging body. Embrace this opportunity to invigorate your life and discover the joy of movement. Your heart, lungs, mind, and spirit will thank you for it.

CHAPTER 2

GETTING STARTED: SAFE CARDIO PRACTICES FOR SENIORS

Embarking on a new exercise routine can be an exciting yet daunting venture, especially for seniors. The key to a successful start lies in understanding the principles of safe cardio practices. This chapter will guide you through the essential steps to ensure your journey into aerobic exercise is both enjoyable and effective.

Consulting with Healthcare Providers

Before diving into any exercise program, it's crucial to consult with your healthcare provider. Medical clearance is a foundational step that can help identify any underlying health issues and establish guidelines tailored to your unique needs. Whether you have chronic conditions, are recovering from an injury, or are simply new to exercise, your doctor can offer valuable insights.

Consider the story of Eleanor, a vibrant 70-year-old who had recently retired. Eager to improve her health, she decided to start a running program. However, her doctor advised against high-impact activities due to a previous knee injury. Instead, he recommended low-impact alternatives, such as walking and cycling, which would still provide cardiovascular benefits without straining her joints. By heeding this advice, Eleanor was able to pursue her fitness goals safely while avoiding potential setbacks.

During your consultation, don't hesitate to discuss any concerns or ask about modifications for specific activities. A healthcare provider can also recommend a physical therapist or a fitness specialist, ensuring you have the right support as you begin your fitness journey.

Listening to Your Body

Once you have medical clearance, the next step is to tune in to your body. As you embark on your cardio routine, it's essential to recognize the signs of fatigue, discomfort, or injury. Many seniors underestimate their bodies' signals, often pushing through pain or fatigue. However, listening to your body is critical to prevent injury and promote a sustainable exercise routine.

Take, for example, the experience of Frank, a 65-year-old who was eager to join a local cycling club. Initially, he felt great and pushed himself to keep up with younger riders. However, he soon developed knee pain. Instead of addressing the discomfort, Frank continued to ride through the pain until it became debilitating. After seeking advice from a physical therapist, he learned the importance of gradual progression and listening to his body's signals. Frank modified his routine, incorporating rest days and adjusting his cycling intensity, allowing him to enjoy the activity without risking injury.

Always pay attention to your energy levels and be mindful of how your body feels during and after workouts. If something doesn't feel right, it's okay to take a step back, modify your routine, or seek professional guidance.

Essential Warm-Up and Cool-Down Routines

Incorporating a proper warm-up and cool-down routine into your workouts is vital for preparing your body and preventing injuries. A warm-up gradually increases your heart rate and warms up your muscles, while a cool-down allows your body to transition back to a resting state.

Before starting your cardio workout, spend 5-10 minutes on a warm-up. This can include gentle movements like arm circles, leg swings, or light walking. For instance, if you plan to go for a brisk walk, begin with a slow stroll to gradually elevate your heart rate and loosen your muscles.

Cool-downs are equally important. After your workout, take 5-10 minutes to perform gentle stretches, focusing on the major muscle groups you engaged during your activity. Not only does this help prevent soreness, but it also enhances flexibility and reduces the risk of injury.

Consider Lisa, a 68-year-old who found joy in water aerobics. She made it a habit to warm up by walking slowly in the shallow end of the pool and incorporated stretching afterward. This practice helped her stay limber and avoided muscle stiffness, allowing her to enjoy her workouts even more.

Creating a Personalized Fitness Plan

With a solid understanding of safe practices, it's time to create a personalized fitness plan. A well-structured plan should take into account your fitness level, health conditions, and personal preferences. Start by assessing your current activity level and any specific goals you wish to achieve.

For example, if you're new to exercise, begin with shorter sessions of low-intensity activities and gradually increase the duration and intensity as you build endurance. Alternatively, if you have specific health concerns, consider exercises that cater to those needs. Your plan might include a mix of activities such as walking, swimming, cycling, or group classes that align with your interests.

Jack, a 72-year-old with a passion for music, decided to incorporate dance aerobics into his routine. With guidance from his doctor, he tailored his plan to include three days of dance classes per week, complemented by two days of brisk walking. By choosing activities he loved, Jack not only stayed committed but also found immense joy in his fitness journey.

As you develop your plan, consider setting achievable goals. Whether it's walking a certain number of steps each day, completing a specific workout, or joining a local fitness class, having clear objectives can keep you motivated. Additionally, regularly revisiting and adjusting your plan as you progress is essential to maintain engagement and challenge yourself.

Starting a cardio routine can be a transformative experience, opening doors to improved health, increased energy, and enhanced quality of life. By consulting with healthcare providers, listening to your body, incorporating warm-up and cool-down routines, and creating a personalized fitness plan, you'll lay the groundwork for a safe and enjoyable journey into aerobic exercise.

As you venture forth, remember the stories of individuals like Eleanor, Frank, Lisa, and Jack—each of whom found success by prioritizing safety and personalization in their fitness journeys. Their experiences serve as reminders that it's never too late to embrace a healthier lifestyle.

In the next chapter, we'll explore various low-impact cardio options that cater specifically to seniors, providing you with a range of enjoyable activities to choose from. Get ready to discover the joy of movement and the countless benefits that await you on your fitness journey!

CHAPTER 3

LOW-IMPACT CARDIO OPTIONS FOR SENIORS

For many seniors, the idea of starting a cardio workout might conjure images of intense training sessions or high-impact exercises that seem daunting. However, low-impact cardio options are abundant and can provide excellent cardiovascular benefits while minimizing the risk of injury. This chapter explores various low-impact activities, making it easier to find the right fit for your lifestyle and preferences.

Walking for Fitness

Walking is often regarded as the simplest and most accessible form of cardio exercise, making it an ideal starting point for seniors. It requires no special equipment, can be done almost anywhere, and is easily adaptable to different fitness levels.

Take the story of Betty, a 74-year-old retiree who discovered the joys of walking in her neighborhood. Initially, she struggled with short distances, but she set a goal to walk around the block each day. Gradually, she increased her distance and even started walking with friends. Before long, Betty found herself looking forward to her daily walks, enjoying both the physical benefits and the social connections they fostered.

To maximize the benefits of walking, focus on maintaining good posture and using a brisk pace that elevates your heart rate without causing strain. Consider joining a walking group or setting specific goals, such as a daily step count, to keep you motivated and accountable.

Water Aerobics

Water aerobics is a gentle yet effective option for seniors, particularly those concerned about joint protection. Exercising in water reduces the impact on your joints, making it an excellent choice for individuals with arthritis or those recovering from injuries. The buoyancy of the water supports your body, allowing for a full range of motion without the stress that comes from exercising on solid ground.

Sarah, a 67-year-old with knee issues, found solace in water aerobics classes at her local community pool. The class was filled with laughter and camaraderie, and she discovered that she could perform movements that felt impossible on land. Over time, Sarah not only improved her cardiovascular endurance but also strengthened her muscles and enhanced her flexibility. Water aerobics became a highlight of her week, combining fitness with social interaction.

If you're interested in water aerobics, look for classes offered at community centers or gyms. Many classes are designed specifically for older adults, focusing on safety and enjoyment while providing a thorough workout.

Cycling & Stationary Bikes

Cycling, whether on a traditional bike or a stationary one, is another fantastic low-impact cardio option. This activity boosts heart rate while protecting the knees and hips, making it suitable for individuals with joint concerns. Riding allows you to control the intensity of your workout, making it adaptable for different fitness levels.

Meet Tom, a 70-year-old who was looking for a way to stay active after a hip replacement. He invested in a stationary bike and started with short sessions while watching his favorite shows. As he built strength and endurance, he gradually increased the duration and intensity of his rides. Tom found that cycling not only improved his cardiovascular health but also offered a fun way to unwind and enjoy his leisure time.

Whether you prefer outdoor cycling or the convenience of a stationary bike, aim for a steady pace that elevates your heart rate. You can also incorporate interval training, alternating between higher and lower intensities, to enhance your workout.

Chair Aerobics

For those with limited mobility or balance issues, chair aerobics provides a safe and effective way to stay active. This form of exercise allows individuals to perform aerobic movements while seated, making it an excellent choice for seniors who may struggle with traditional workouts.

Joan, an 80-year-old with balance challenges, found chair aerobics to be a perfect solution. She joined a local class where participants engaged in rhythmic movements while seated. Joan loved the upbeat music and the sense of community among her fellow participants. Over time, she noticed increased energy levels and improved overall strength.

Chair aerobics can be tailored to your specific needs, allowing you to incorporate upper-body movements, leg lifts, and even stretching while seated. Look for classes in your area or find online resources to guide you through chair-based workouts.

Tai Chi and Dance

Tai Chi and dance are excellent low-impact activities that not only promote cardiovascular endurance but also improve coordination and balance. Both forms of exercise encourage fluid movements, helping to enhance flexibility and stability.

Linda, a 66-year-old former dancer, rediscovered her love for movement by joining a local Tai Chi class. The gentle flowing motions helped her develop better balance and reduce stress, all while getting her heart rate up. She found that Tai Chi not only improved her physical health but also provided a calming routine that centered her mind.

Similarly, dance classes—whether it's ballroom, line dancing, or even Zumba Gold—offer a joyful way to engage in aerobic exercise. George, who had always loved to dance, joined a weekly class that catered to seniors. He found that dancing brought back cherished memories while providing a fun cardiovascular workout.

Both Tai Chi and dance classes often foster a sense of community, making them ideal for social interaction while promoting physical health. Check local community centers or dance studios for offerings tailored to seniors.

Exploring low-impact cardio options can lead to a fulfilling and enjoyable fitness journey. From walking and water aerobics to cycling, chair aerobics, Tai Chi, and dance, there's something for everyone. The stories of Betty, Sarah, Tom, Joan, and Linda illustrate the diverse ways seniors can stay active while prioritizing safety and enjoyment.

As you consider which activities resonate with you, remember that the most important aspect of any exercise routine is finding something you love. When you enjoy your workouts, you're more likely to stick with them, reaping the myriad benefits of cardiovascular health and overall well-being.

In the next chapter, we'll delve into creating a supportive environment for your fitness journey, including finding community resources, motivation, and ways to stay accountable. Embrace the joy of movement as we continue this adventure toward a healthier, more active life!

CHAPTER 4

GOLDEN AEROBICS ROUTINES FOR ACTIVE SENIORS

As we delve deeper into the world of aerobic exercise, it's essential to explore routines specifically designed for active seniors. These routines not only enhance cardiovascular health but also focus on building stamina and keeping workouts enjoyable. In this chapter, we'll cover moderate-intensity cardio workouts, interval training, step aerobics, dance-based workouts, and Nordic walking—each offering unique benefits tailored to older adults.

Moderate-Intensity Cardio Workouts

Moderate-intensity cardio workouts are a fantastic way for seniors to build stamina without straining the body. These workouts can be easily adjusted to match individual fitness levels while promoting heart health and overall endurance.

Consider Margaret, a 68-year-old who decided to start a walking program. She began by walking briskly for 20 minutes, focusing on maintaining a pace that elevated her heart rate but still allowed her to hold a conversation. Over the weeks, Margaret gradually increased her walking time to 30 minutes, adding variety by exploring different routes in her neighborhood. The moderate-intensity of her walks improved her cardiovascular fitness, and she found herself enjoying the fresh air and the sights around her.

To incorporate moderate-intensity cardio into your routine, aim for activities like brisk walking, swimming at a steady pace, or cycling on flat terrain. The goal is to reach a level of exertion where you can talk but not sing—a good indicator of moderate intensity. Aim for at least 150 minutes of moderate-intensity cardio each week, broken down into manageable sessions.

Interval Training for Seniors

Interval training involves alternating periods of higher intensity with periods of lower intensity or rest. This method can be especially beneficial for seniors, as it helps build endurance and strength without requiring prolonged exertion.

Take John, a 72-year-old who was looking for a way to spice up his walking routine. With the guidance of a fitness coach, he started incorporating intervals into his walks. John would walk briskly for two minutes, then slow down to a moderate pace for one minute, repeating this cycle for 30 minutes. This simple adjustment made his workouts more dynamic and engaging.

Interval training can be applied to various activities, such as walking, cycling, or even water aerobics. The key is to find a balance that feels comfortable yet challenging. Start with short intervals, like 20 seconds of higher intensity followed by a minute of lower intensity, gradually increasing the length of your higher-intensity bursts as you build fitness. This method not only enhances cardiovascular fitness but also improves metabolic health, helping with weight management.

Step Aerobics & Dance-Based Workouts

Step aerobics and dance-based workouts offer a fun, rhythmic way to engage in cardio exercise while improving coordination and balance. These workouts are perfect for seniors looking for an enjoyable way to stay active.

Nancy, a lively 75-year-old, joined a step aerobics class at her local community center. She was initially nervous but soon found herself immersed in the energetic atmosphere. The instructor led the class through a series of choreographed movements, incorporating a step platform that added variety and intensity. Nancy loved the music and the sense of community that the class provided. Over time, she noticed improved balance and coordination, as well as a significant boost in her cardiovascular fitness.

Dance-based workouts, such as Zumba Gold or line dancing, also provide excellent opportunities to enjoy movement while getting a workout. These classes are designed with seniors in mind, featuring lower-impact choreography that encourages participants to move at their own pace. George, who joined a Zumba Gold class, discovered that dancing allowed him to express himself while also working up a sweat. The combination of fun music and social interaction kept him motivated and engaged.

When participating in step aerobics or dance classes, choose a pace that feels comfortable. These workouts can be easily adapted to individual fitness levels, allowing you to progress as your stamina improves.

Nordic Walking

Nordic walking is an excellent way to increase the intensity of your cardio workouts while engaging the entire body. This technique involves using specially designed poles that help propel you forward, providing a full-body workout that enhances cardiovascular health and builds strength.

Consider Clara, a 70-year-old who wanted to add variety to her fitness routine. After learning about Nordic walking from a friend, she decided to join a local group. With the guidance of an instructor, Clara learned how to use the poles effectively, which not only improved her balance but also engaged her arms and core during her walks. As she became more comfortable with the technique, Clara found that her walks became more dynamic and enjoyable.

Nordic walking is beneficial for seniors as it reduces the impact on joints while increasing calorie burn. It's particularly useful for those looking to strengthen their upper body and improve cardiovascular fitness simultaneously. If you're interested in trying Nordic walking, consider joining a class or finding a tutorial online to learn proper technique. Look for lightweight, adjustable poles designed specifically for this activity.

Putting It All Together: Crafting Your Routine

As you explore these various aerobic options, it's essential to remember that consistency is key. Incorporating a variety of activities can keep your routine fresh and enjoyable while targeting different muscle groups and cardiovascular systems.

When crafting your routine, consider mixing moderate-intensity workouts with interval training sessions, step aerobics or dance classes, and Nordic walking. For example, you might plan:

- Monday: Moderate-intensity walking for 30 minutes.

- Wednesday: Step aerobics class for 45 minutes.

- Friday: Interval training walk, alternating brisk and moderate paces for 30 minutes.

- Saturday: Nordic walking with a group for 60 minutes.

Make sure to listen to your body and adjust the intensity and duration of your workouts as needed. Always include warm-up and cool-down routines to prepare your body for exercise and aid in recovery.

Enjoying the Journey

The variety of aerobic options available for seniors ensures that there's something for everyone, whether you prefer the simplicity of walking or the dynamic energy of dance-based workouts. The stories of Margaret, John, Nancy, Clara, and George highlight the diverse ways seniors can embrace fitness while enjoying the process.

As you embark on your own golden aerobics journey, remember that the most important aspect is to find activities that resonate with you and bring you joy. The more you enjoy your workouts, the more likely you are to stick with them, paving the way for a healthier, more active lifestyle.

In the next chapter, we will discuss the importance of nutrition and hydration in supporting your cardio workouts and overall health. Get ready to discover how nourishing your body can enhance your fitness journey and well-being!

CHAPTER 5

MANAGING AGE-RELATED CHALLENGES DURING CARDIO WORKOUTS

As we age, our bodies naturally encounter various challenges that can affect our ability to engage in physical activity. However, with the right strategies and modifications, these challenges can be effectively managed, allowing seniors to enjoy the benefits of cardio workouts safely and comfortably. In this chapter, we'll explore how to adapt to conditions like arthritis, joint pain, or osteoporosis, modify routines for heart conditions, maintain balance and safety, and utilize breathing techniques to enhance endurance.

Adapting to Arthritis, Joint Pain, or Osteoporosis

Arthritis, joint pain, and osteoporosis are common age-related conditions that can make traditional workouts uncomfortable or even risky. However, adapting your cardio routine can significantly improve mobility and strength while minimizing discomfort.

For example, consider Elaine, a 71-year-old who had been living with osteoarthritis in her knees. She initially hesitated to exercise, fearing it would worsen her pain. However, after consulting with her doctor and a physical therapist, Elaine discovered low-impact activities that would allow her to stay active. She started with water aerobics, where the buoyancy of the water reduced strain on her joints while providing resistance for muscle strengthening. Over time, Elaine became more confident in her abilities and began incorporating gentle cycling into her routine.

When managing arthritis or joint pain, it's essential to choose safe workouts that promote flexibility and strength. Here are some strategies:

1. Focus on Low-Impact Activities: Swimming, cycling, and walking are excellent options that minimize stress on joints. These activities allow for cardiovascular benefits without exacerbating pain.

2. Incorporate Strength Training: Building muscle can help support joints and improve overall stability. Light resistance training, using bands or light weights, can enhance strength without causing discomfort.

3. Warm-Up and Stretch: Always begin with a thorough warm-up to prepare your joints for movement. Gentle stretching can improve flexibility and reduce stiffness.

4. Listen to Your Body: Pay attention to any signs of discomfort and adjust your workouts accordingly. If a particular movement causes pain, it's important to modify or avoid it.

Cardio for Heart Conditions

For seniors with cardiovascular health issues, managing exercise routines is crucial. While physical activity is essential for heart health, modifications may be necessary to ensure safety and effectiveness.

Take the story of Robert, a 75-year-old who had undergone heart surgery a year prior. He was eager to return to exercise but was unsure how to approach it safely. After working closely with his cardiologist and a rehabilitation specialist, Robert learned how to modify his cardio workouts. He began with short walks on flat surfaces, gradually increasing duration and intensity as recommended by his healthcare team.

When exercising with a heart condition, consider the following tips:

1. Consult Your Healthcare Provider: Before starting any new workout regimen, it's essential to seek medical advice. Your doctor can provide personalized recommendations based on your specific condition and fitness level.

2. Start Slow: Gradually ease into your routine, focusing on short sessions of low-intensity activities. As your fitness improves, you can incrementally increase duration and intensity.

3. Monitor Your Heart Rate: Keeping track of your heart rate during workouts can help you stay within safe limits. Your healthcare provider can guide you on target heart rate zones that are appropriate for your condition.

4. Choose Activities Wisely: Opt for low-impact exercises that minimize strain on the heart, such as walking, cycling, or using a recumbent bike. These activities can enhance cardiovascular fitness without overexerting your heart.

5. Stay Hydrated and Nourished: Proper hydration and nutrition are essential for heart health. Ensure you're drinking enough water and consuming a balanced diet rich in fruits, vegetables, whole grains, and lean proteins.

Balancing Mobility and Safety

Maintaining balance and safety during aerobic exercises is paramount, particularly for seniors who may be concerned about falls or instability. It's important to adopt strategies that promote confidence and steadiness while engaging in cardio workouts.

Consider Helen, an 80-year-old who loved to walk but had experienced a few near-falls due to balance issues. Determined to stay active, she sought advice from a physical therapist, who taught her techniques to improve her stability. Helen learned to engage her core muscles and focus on her foot placement during walks, which significantly boosted her confidence.

Here are some effective strategies for enhancing balance and safety during workouts:

1. **Use Supportive Gear:** Wear well-fitting shoes with good grip to prevent slipping. If necessary, consider using a cane or walking poles for added support.

2. **Engage Your Core:** Strengthening your core muscles can enhance overall stability. Incorporate exercises like seated leg lifts or gentle abdominal contractions into your routine.

3. **Focus on Controlled Movements**: Perform exercises slowly and deliberately to maintain control. Avoid rapid, jerky motions that can increase the risk of losing balance.

4. **Choose Safe Environments:** When exercising, opt for well-lit and flat areas. Avoid uneven terrain and crowded spaces to minimize the risk of accidents.

5. Practice Balance Exercises: Incorporate specific balance training into your routine, such as standing on one foot or using a balance board. These exercises can enhance your stability and confidence.

6. Workout with a Buddy: Exercising with a friend or family member can provide extra support and motivation. It also creates a safety net in case of any unexpected falls.

Breathing Techniques & Endurance

Maximizing oxygen flow is crucial for improving endurance during cardio workouts. Learning proper breathing techniques can enhance performance and make exercise feel easier and more enjoyable.

Take the example of Steve, a 69-year-old who struggled with breathlessness during workouts. Frustrated, he decided to take a yoga class focused on breathing techniques. He learned to incorporate deep, diaphragmatic breathing into his exercise routine, which allowed for better oxygen intake. Over time, Steve noticed a significant improvement in his endurance and overall comfort during workouts.

To enhance your breathing and endurance during cardio exercises, consider the following techniques:

1. Practice Deep Breathing: Focus on breathing deeply from your diaphragm rather than shallowly from your chest. Inhale through your nose, allowing your belly to rise, and exhale through your mouth, letting your belly fall.

2. Establish a Breathing Rhythm: Coordinate your breath with your movements. For example, inhale for a count of two during exertion and exhale for a count of three during recovery. This rhythm can help maintain steady oxygen flow.

3. Incorporate Breathing Exercises: Spend a few minutes each day practicing breathing exercises. Try inhaling for a count of four, holding for four, and exhaling for four. This practice can help train your lungs and improve overall endurance.

4. Stay Relaxed: Tension can restrict breathing. Focus on staying relaxed and maintaining good posture during workouts to allow for optimal oxygen flow.

5. Gradually Increase Workout Duration: As you improve your breathing techniques, gradually extend the duration of your workouts. This progression can help enhance your overall cardiovascular endurance.

Overcoming Challenges with Resilience

Managing age-related challenges during cardio workouts doesn't have to be an obstacle; instead, it can be an opportunity for growth and resilience. The stories of Elaine, Robert, Helen, and Steve illustrate how seniors can adapt their routines to stay active and healthy despite various limitations.

By focusing on safe adaptations for conditions like arthritis and heart issues, maintaining balance and safety, and utilizing effective breathing techniques, seniors can continue to enjoy the myriad benefits of aerobic exercise. Remember that every small step you take contributes to your overall well-being and vitality.

In the next chapter, we will explore the role of nutrition in supporting your cardio workouts, highlighting the best foods and hydration strategies to fuel your body for optimal performance. Get ready to discover how nourishing your body can enhance your fitness journey!

CHAPTER 6

CARDIO WORKOUTS TO BOOST COGNITIVE FUNCTION

As we navigate the later stages of life, the importance of maintaining not just physical health but also cognitive function becomes paramount. Studies increasingly show that aerobic exercise plays a significant role in preserving brain health, enhancing memory, and fostering social connections—all essential components for a fulfilling life. In this chapter, we'll explore the connection between cardio and brain health, specific aerobic activities that bolster cognitive function, and the benefits of group fitness classes for social engagement.

The Connection Between Cardio and Brain Health

The relationship between physical activity and brain health has been a focal point of research for years. Numerous studies suggest that engaging in regular aerobic exercise can significantly reduce the risk of dementia and cognitive decline. But how does this work?

Consider the case of Doris, a vibrant 76-year-old who has always prioritized her fitness. After reading about the benefits of cardio for brain health, she became even more committed to her routine, engaging in activities like brisk walking and swimming several times a week. Doris was intrigued by the science behind these benefits, so she began attending workshops and reading research articles on the topic.

One of the key findings is that aerobic exercise increases blood flow to the brain, providing essential nutrients and oxygen that support neuronal health. Moreover, exercise promotes the release of growth factors, such as brain-derived neurotrophic factor (BDNF), which encourages the growth and survival of neurons.

Additionally, physical activity can help reduce inflammation and oxidative stress—two factors that have been linked to cognitive decline. The more active Doris became, the more she felt mentally alert and focused, noticing a positive change in her ability to concentrate on tasks and remember details.

To harness the brain-boosting benefits of cardio, aim for at least 150 minutes of moderate-intensity aerobic activity each week. Whether it's walking, cycling, or swimming, regular engagement in these activities can significantly contribute to cognitive resilience as you age.

Aerobic Activity for Memory and Focus

While all aerobic exercises offer benefits for brain health, some specific activities are particularly effective at supporting memory and focus. Let's explore a few of these engaging workouts.

1. Walking and Hiking

Walking is perhaps the most accessible form of aerobic exercise, and it comes with numerous cognitive benefits. Studies show that just a brisk walk can improve memory performance and enhance focus. For instance, when Martha, a 65-year-old grandmother, started walking in her neighborhood three times a week, she noticed that not only did her mood improve, but her ability to recall names and faces also sharpened.

Adding nature to the mix, like hiking in a local park, can enhance these benefits even further. The combination of physical exertion and exposure to natural environments has been shown to reduce stress and improve cognitive function.

2. Dancing

Dance-based workouts offer a dual benefit: physical activity and mental stimulation. Engaging in dance requires coordination, memory, and concentration—all of which challenge the brain. For example, after joining a local dance class, 70-year-old Tom found that learning new routines improved his cognitive skills. The rhythmic movements and social aspects of dancing provided both a workout and a mental challenge.

Studies have demonstrated that dance can enhance neuroplasticity—the brain's ability to form new connections—leading to improved memory and cognitive flexibility. So whether you prefer ballroom dancing, Zumba, or line dancing, this lively workout can significantly boost brain health.

3. Cycling

Cycling, whether on a stationary bike or outdoors, is another excellent cardio option. It enhances cardiovascular fitness while also improving attention and concentration. Lucy, a retired teacher, took up cycling to explore her local trails. Not only did she enjoy the physical benefits, but she also found that her mental clarity improved, making it easier to engage in her favorite hobby: reading.

Research indicates that aerobic activities like cycling can stimulate the production of BDNF, fostering the growth of new brain cells. This, in turn, may help improve memory retention and cognitive performance, making cycling a fantastic choice for brain health.

Group Fitness Classes for Social Engagement

Beyond the physical and cognitive benefits, group fitness classes offer an invaluable opportunity for social engagement. Social interaction is vital for mental health and can enhance cognitive function. When seniors come together to exercise, they create a sense of community and support that contributes to overall well-being.

Take, for example, the story of Elaine and her friends. After retiring, Elaine wanted to stay active and connected with others, so she joined a weekly aerobics class at the local community center. The class not only provided a structured workout but also fostered friendships. The laughter, shared stories, and mutual encouragement created an uplifting atmosphere that benefited everyone involved.

1. Building Relationships

The social aspect of group classes encourages interaction and camaraderie. As Elaine and her friends navigated challenging routines together, they supported one another, creating bonds that extended beyond the exercise floor. Studies have shown that strong social ties can reduce the risk of cognitive decline, highlighting the importance of community in maintaining brain health.

2. Teamwork and Cooperation

Group classes often incorporate elements of teamwork, whether it's through partner exercises or group challenges. This cooperative environment stimulates cognitive function as participants strategize and communicate. Tom, who initially hesitated to join a group, found that participating in team-based activities not only improved his fitness but also sharpened his decision-making skills as he worked alongside others.

3. Structured Learning

In a group setting, participants often have access to knowledgeable instructors who can provide guidance and modifications tailored to different fitness levels. This structured learning environment enhances the overall workout experience and allows seniors to push their boundaries in a safe, supportive space.

Tips for Incorporating Cardio to Boost Cognitive Function

1. Start Small: If you're new to exercise, begin with short sessions and gradually increase your duration and intensity. Even short bursts of activity can have a positive impact on brain health.

2. Mix It Up: Incorporate a variety of aerobic activities into your routine to keep it fresh and engaging. Try walking one day, dancing the next, and perhaps cycling on the weekends.

3. Stay Social: Join a class or find a workout buddy to enhance your motivation and enjoyment. The social interactions will enrich your experience and provide additional cognitive benefits.

4. Set Goals: Establishing fitness goals can keep you motivated and engaged. Whether it's completing a certain number of classes each month or increasing your walking distance, goals can provide direction and purpose.

5. Keep It Fun: Choose activities that you genuinely enjoy. When you have fun, you're more likely to stick with your routine, ensuring you reap the cognitive benefits of regular cardio exercise.

A Holistic Approach to Brain Health

The profound connection between cardio workouts and cognitive function underscores the importance of integrating physical activity into daily life, particularly as we age. Through engaging in aerobic exercises like walking, dancing, and cycling, seniors can enhance memory, improve focus, and fortify their mental resilience.

The stories of Doris, Martha, Tom, and Elaine illustrate the transformative power of exercise—not just for physical health, but for cognitive vitality and social well-being. By embracing a holistic approach that incorporates movement and community, you can cultivate a lifestyle that nurtures both the body and the mind.

In the next chapter, we will explore the importance of recovery and rest in your cardio regimen, ensuring that you maintain a balanced approach to fitness and overall health. Prepare to discover how proper recovery can enhance your performance and longevity in your exercise journey!

CHAPTER 7

NUTRITION AND RECOVERY FOR SENIOR CARDIO ENTHUSIASTS

As we embrace an active lifestyle, particularly through cardio workouts, understanding the vital role of nutrition and recovery becomes essential. Proper nutrition not only fuels our bodies for exercise but also supports heart health and overall well-being. Additionally, effective recovery strategies ensure we maintain our fitness levels while preventing injury and promoting longevity. In this chapter, we'll explore optimal nutrition for seniors, hydration strategies, and the importance of muscle recovery and rest.

Fueling the Aging Body

As we age, our nutritional needs change. For seniors, focusing on heart-healthy foods that provide sustained energy and support cardiovascular function is critical. Let's dive into the types of nutrients that can enhance your performance and overall health.

1. Prioritizing Whole Foods

The foundation of a nutritious diet should be whole foods—fruits, vegetables, whole grains, lean proteins, and healthy fats. Consider the journey of George, an 82-year-old who recently made a commitment to improve his eating habits. After attending a local workshop on nutrition, he learned about the benefits of incorporating more fruits and vegetables into his meals. George began filling his plate with vibrant salads and roasted veggies, feeling more energized during his cardio sessions.

Whole foods are packed with essential vitamins, minerals, and antioxidants that help reduce inflammation and support heart health. Aim for a colorful variety to maximize nutrient intake, ensuring you get a broad spectrum of health benefits.

2. Lean Proteins for Muscle Maintenance

As we age, maintaining muscle mass becomes increasingly important. Including adequate protein in your diet supports muscle repair and growth, especially after cardio workouts. Sources of lean protein include chicken, fish, beans, lentils, and low-fat dairy products.

Take, for example, Linda, a 70-year-old grandmother who enjoys cycling. After learning about protein's importance for recovery, she began adding Greek yogurt and nuts to her post-workout snacks. This change not only aided her recovery but also helped her feel stronger and more capable during her rides.

3. Healthy Fats for Energy

Incorporating healthy fats into your diet can provide a sustained source of energy for your cardio workouts. Foods such as avocados, nuts, seeds, and olive oil are excellent choices. For instance, Richard, a 75-year-old who enjoys brisk walking, found that adding a handful of walnuts to his morning oatmeal kept him feeling full and energized throughout his walks.

Healthy fats also support heart health by improving cholesterol levels and reducing inflammation, making them a crucial part of a balanced diet.

4. Carbohydrates for Fuel

While it's important to focus on quality carbohydrates, they should not be overlooked, especially for those engaging in regular cardio. Whole grains, fruits, and vegetables provide the energy needed to fuel your workouts. Consider Sarah, a 68-year-old who loves to dance. She discovered that including whole grain toast or oatmeal before her dance classes provided the energy she needed to keep up with the routines.

Aim for complex carbohydrates that digest slowly, providing steady energy throughout your activities. This approach will help maintain your stamina during workouts and support overall health.

Hydration Tips for Seniors

Staying properly hydrated is crucial for everyone, but it becomes even more important as we age. Dehydration can lead to fatigue, dizziness, and decreased performance, making hydration a key component of your fitness routine.

1. The Importance of Hydration

Our bodies are composed of around 60% water, and maintaining hydration is essential for numerous bodily functions, including temperature regulation, joint lubrication, and nutrient transport. Seniors may be at a higher risk for dehydration due to changes in thirst perception and kidney function.

Joan, a 72-year-old who enjoys morning walks, learned the importance of hydration the hard way. After feeling unusually fatigued during her walks, she discovered she hadn't been drinking enough water. Once she started keeping a water bottle with her and sipping regularly, her energy levels and overall enjoyment of her walks improved dramatically.

2. Hydration Before, During, and After Workouts

- Before Workouts: Aim to drink water before exercising to ensure your body is well-hydrated. A good rule of thumb is to drink about 8 ounces of water 30 minutes prior to your workout.

- During Workouts: If your workout lasts longer than 30 minutes, consider sipping water at regular intervals. For activities lasting over an hour, sports drinks with electrolytes can help replenish lost minerals.

- After Workouts: Rehydrate post-exercise to help with recovery. Drinking water or an electrolyte-rich beverage can aid in muscle repair and overall recovery.

3. Recognizing Signs of Dehydration

Being aware of the signs of dehydration is essential. Common symptoms include dry mouth, fatigue, dizziness, and dark urine. To prevent dehydration, make it a habit to check in with your body regularly, especially during and after physical activity.

Muscle Recovery and Rest

While cardio is vital for cardiovascular health and overall fitness, recovery and rest are equally important. Giving your body time to recuperate allows muscles to repair and grow stronger, preventing burnout and injury.

1. The Importance of Recovery

After an intense cardio session, your body needs time to recover. This is when muscles repair and adapt, allowing for improved performance in future workouts.

Tom, who loves to jog, learned about the importance of recovery after pushing himself too hard during training. He noticed he was feeling fatigued and not making progress. By incorporating rest days and lighter activity days into his routine, he found his energy levels rebounded, and he enjoyed his runs much more.

2. Active Recovery Techniques

Active recovery refers to low-intensity activities performed on rest days. This can include leisurely walking, gentle stretching, or yoga. For instance, Helen, a 76-year-old who participates in group aerobics, incorporates yoga on her rest days. This practice not only aids in muscle recovery but also enhances flexibility and relaxation.

3. Sleep: The Ultimate Recovery Tool

Never underestimate the power of a good night's sleep. Sleep plays a crucial role in recovery, allowing your body to repair itself and regulate hormones that influence appetite and stress. Aim for 7-9 hours of quality sleep each night.

Mark, a 69-year-old who struggled with sleep quality, found that establishing a bedtime routine helped him achieve better rest. By going to bed at the same time each night and creating a calming environment, he improved his sleep quality, leading to more energy and better performance in his cardio workouts.

4. Stretching and Mobility Work

Incorporating stretching and mobility work into your routine can enhance recovery by improving flexibility and reducing muscle tightness. Simple stretches post-workout can promote blood flow and help prevent soreness.

After her cardio sessions, Anne, a 73-year-old who loves cycling, dedicates time to stretching her legs and back. This practice has made her feel more agile and has significantly reduced post-exercise soreness.

Nutrition and recovery are foundational elements of a successful fitness journey, especially for senior cardio enthusiasts. By fueling your body with the right foods, staying properly hydrated, and prioritizing recovery, you can enhance your workouts and overall health.

The stories of George, Linda, Richard, Joan, and others highlight how mindful choices in nutrition and recovery can lead to improved performance, increased energy, and a more enjoyable fitness experience.

As you embrace your cardio journey, remember that taking care of your body through proper nutrition and recovery is just as important as the workouts themselves. In the next chapter, we'll explore how to set achievable fitness goals and maintain motivation on your path to lifelong health and wellness. Get ready to unlock your potential!

CHAPTER 8

CREATING LONG-TERM CARDIO HABITS

Establishing a sustainable fitness routine is essential for reaping the benefits of cardio exercise, especially as we age. The journey to long-term cardio habits involves finding motivation, tracking progress, adding variety to your workouts, and overcoming obstacles along the way. This chapter will provide insights and practical strategies to help you create lasting cardio habits that enhance your physical and mental well-being.

Staying Motivated with Routine

Motivation can ebb and flow, but establishing a consistent routine can help you stay committed to your cardio workouts. Let's explore how to build a sustainable routine that fits into your lifestyle.

1. Setting a Schedule

Just like any important appointment, schedule your workouts as part of your weekly agenda. Consider Martha, a 65-year-old who recently retired. She decided to reserve her mornings for cardio, treating them as sacred "me time." By setting specific days and times for her walks, she created a reliable routine that became part of her daily life.

This commitment made it easier for her to stay on track. She learned to prioritize these sessions, finding that they not only boosted her physical health but also improved her mood and energy levels.

2. Find Your "Why"

Identifying your personal motivations can significantly enhance your commitment. Whether it's improving heart health, maintaining independence, or simply feeling good, knowing why you exercise can drive you to stick with it. Richard, for example, discovered that his motivation stemmed from wanting to keep up with his grandchildren. This realization fueled his dedication to regular walking and cycling, making every session feel purposeful.

3. Build a Support System

Engaging family and friends can provide an extra layer of motivation. Consider Linda, who invited a friend to join her for weekly dance classes. Not only did this make the workouts more enjoyable, but it also created accountability. When her friend couldn't make it, Linda found that she still pushed herself to go, knowing that her friend would be eager to hear about her experience.

Tracking Progress

Monitoring your progress is a powerful way to maintain motivation and see how far you've come. Tracking can take many forms, and finding what works for you can help you celebrate your achievements.

1. Measuring Heart Rate

One effective way to track progress is by monitoring your heart rate during workouts. This can provide insight into your cardiovascular fitness and help you understand how your body responds to exercise. For example, Tom invested in a simple heart rate monitor, which he wore during his runs. Over time, he noticed that his heart rate during the same intensity level decreased, indicating improved cardiovascular health. This tangible evidence of progress motivated him to continue his training.

2. Endurance and Distance Goals

Setting specific endurance or distance goals can also be beneficial. For example, George, who enjoyed walking, aimed to increase his distance from one mile to two. He documented his walks in a journal, noting not just the distance but also how he felt during each session. This method not only tracked his progress but also provided insights into his energy levels, allowing him to adjust his routine as needed.

3. Celebrate Small Victories

Recognizing small milestones along the way can boost your motivation. If you've increased your walking speed, completed a new route, or managed to engage in a longer workout, celebrate these achievements! Linda rewarded herself with a new pair of workout shoes when she reached her goal of consistently exercising three times a week. These celebrations create positive reinforcement, encouraging you to keep going.

Incorporating Fun and Variety

Keeping your cardio routine exciting and enjoyable is essential for long-term adherence. Boredom can quickly lead to a lack of motivation, so finding ways to mix things up will keep you engaged.

1. Explore New Activities

Experimenting with different forms of cardio can add excitement to your routine. For example, while cycling is fantastic for cardiovascular fitness, Richard decided to try kayaking with a local group. This new activity not only provided a fresh challenge but also introduced him to new friends who shared his passion for the outdoors.

Consider joining a group class or trying a new activity each month. Whether it's a dance class, swimming, or hiking, these experiences can invigorate your routine and keep you motivated.

2. Make It Social

Integrating social elements into your workouts can also enhance enjoyment. Group activities often provide a sense of community that makes exercise more enjoyable. For instance, Joan organized a walking group in her neighborhood, inviting neighbors to join her twice a week. The laughter and camaraderie transformed their walks into a social event, making them something to look forward to rather than just another workout.

3. Use Technology for Variety

Embrace technology to keep your workouts fresh. Fitness apps and online videos offer a plethora of options for different workout styles and intensities. Helen discovered an app with guided dance workouts and began exploring various routines from the comfort of her living room. This not only kept her cardio exciting but also allowed her to learn new moves at her own pace.

Overcoming Plateaus

As you progress in your fitness journey, you may encounter plateaus—periods where you feel like your progress has stalled. Understanding how to adjust your routines can help you overcome these challenges and continue making gains.

1. Mix Up Your Routine

If you find yourself hitting a plateau, it may be time to change your workout routine. This doesn't necessarily mean starting from scratch; small adjustments can reignite progress. For instance, if you've been walking the same route at the same pace, try increasing your speed, adding intervals, or exploring new trails. Tom, for example, found that incorporating short bursts of jogging into his walks helped him break through a fitness plateau, enhancing both his stamina and enjoyment.

2. Increase Intensity Gradually

Gradually increasing the intensity of your workouts can also help combat plateaus. If you've been exercising at a moderate level, consider adding short intervals of higher intensity or extending your workout duration. George started incorporating hill workouts into his walking routine, which not only challenged him but also led to noticeable improvements in his endurance.

3. Seek Professional Guidance

If you're unsure how to adjust your routine, consider consulting a fitness professional. A trainer can assess your current fitness level and provide personalized recommendations to help you continue progressing. Linda decided to work with a trainer for a few sessions, gaining valuable insights into new exercises and modifications that kept her motivated and on track.

Creating long-term cardio habits is a journey that involves motivation, tracking, variety, and adaptability. By developing a consistent routine, monitoring your progress, incorporating fun activities, and learning how to overcome plateaus, you can foster a sustainable cardio lifestyle that enhances your health and vitality as you age.

The stories of Martha, Richard, Tom, Linda, and Joan illustrate the power of commitment and creativity in building lasting fitness habits. As you embark on your journey, remember that every step counts, and finding joy in your activities is essential.

In the next chapter, we'll delve into the importance of setting achievable fitness goals and maintaining motivation throughout your journey. Get ready to unlock your potential and embrace a healthier, more active lifestyle!

CHAPTER 9

CARDIO WORKOUTS FOR SPECIAL POPULATIONS

Incorporating cardio workouts into daily life is essential for everyone, but for certain populations, tailored approaches are necessary to ensure safety and effectiveness. Seniors with diabetes, respiratory conditions, or limited mobility face unique challenges, yet with the right strategies and modifications, they can reap the benefits of aerobic exercise. This chapter explores cardio options specifically designed for these groups, providing practical advice and inspiring stories along the way.

Cardio for Seniors with Diabetes

For seniors living with diabetes, maintaining stable blood sugar levels is a top priority. Regular aerobic exercise can play a pivotal role in managing diabetes effectively, helping to enhance insulin sensitivity and promote overall health.

1. Understanding the Benefits

Engaging in regular cardio can help seniors with diabetes lower their blood sugar levels and improve their overall cardiovascular health. Research has shown that even moderate-intensity aerobic activities, such as brisk walking, can significantly impact glucose control. For instance, when Samuel, a 70-year-old retiree diagnosed with type 2 diabetes, began a routine of daily walks, he noticed a remarkable difference in his blood sugar readings. Not only did his levels stabilize, but he also felt more energized throughout the day.

2. Creating a Safe Routine

Before starting any exercise program, seniors with diabetes should consult their healthcare provider. This ensures they receive tailored advice based on their medical history. Monitoring blood sugar levels before and after workouts is essential. This practice helps determine how exercise affects individual glucose levels, allowing for better management and adjustments to diet and medication if necessary.

For Samuel, carrying a glucose monitor during his walks became a crucial part of his routine. He learned to recognize the signs of low blood sugar and how to respond effectively. After a few weeks of consistent walking, he felt more in control of his health and began to experiment with longer walks, finding joy in exploring local parks.

3. Incorporating Aerobic Activities

Seniors with diabetes can benefit from various aerobic activities beyond walking. Swimming, cycling, and group fitness classes can all contribute to improved health outcomes. Sarah, an active 68-year-old with diabetes, discovered water aerobics through a local community center. The low-impact nature of the class allowed her to exercise without stressing her joints, all while enjoying the camaraderie of others facing similar health challenges.

Water aerobics not only provided cardiovascular benefits but also helped her manage her weight and improve her mood. The buoyancy of the water made every movement feel easier, making her more likely to stick with her routine.

Cardio for Seniors with Respiratory Conditions

Seniors with respiratory conditions, such as asthma or chronic obstructive pulmonary disease (COPD), may find cardio workouts daunting. However, with the right approach, they can safely engage in aerobic activities that promote lung health and overall fitness.

1. Breathing Techniques for Better Performance

Understanding how to breathe effectively is vital for seniors with respiratory issues. Incorporating specific breathing techniques can help improve lung function and endurance. For example, using diaphragmatic breathing—focusing on deep, abdominal breaths—can enhance oxygen intake and reduce breathlessness.

Take, for instance, Helen, a 72-year-old diagnosed with COPD. Before beginning her cardio journey, she consulted a respiratory therapist, who taught her various breathing techniques. By practicing these techniques during her walking sessions, she became more aware of her breathing patterns, learning to take deeper, more controlled breaths that improved her stamina.

2. Choosing Suitable Activities

Low-impact aerobic exercises are ideal for seniors with respiratory conditions. Walking at a comfortable pace, swimming, and stationary cycling are excellent choices. These activities can be easily adjusted to accommodate energy levels and lung capacity.

Helen discovered that joining a walking group was both motivational and supportive. Having others around made it easier to push through challenging moments, and she felt encouraged by the shared experience. As her fitness improved, she gradually increased her walking duration, celebrating each milestone with her new friends.

3. Monitoring and Adjusting

Seniors with respiratory conditions should continuously monitor their breathing during workouts. It's essential to start slow and gradually increase intensity based on comfort levels. Joan, a 69-year-old with asthma, learned to carry her inhaler during her fitness sessions. By starting with short walks and gradually increasing her pace and distance, she was able to enjoy the fresh air without triggering her asthma.

Joan also became adept at recognizing her body's signals. She learned to take breaks when needed, allowing herself time to catch her breath and stay safe while still benefiting from her cardio routine.

For Seniors with Limited Mobility

For seniors with limited mobility, traditional cardio workouts may not be feasible. However, there are numerous adaptive cardio options that can promote cardiovascular health without compromising safety.

1. Chair Exercises

Chair exercises are an excellent way for seniors with limited mobility to stay active. These exercises can be tailored to individual needs and can be performed from the comfort of a chair. Simple movements like seated leg lifts, arm raises, and gentle twists can provide cardiovascular benefits while ensuring safety.

Consider George, a 75-year-old who suffered a knee injury that limited his mobility. With the help of a physical therapist, he discovered a series of chair exercises that allowed him to engage in cardio without putting pressure on his knee. He found that these exercises not only elevated his heart rate but also improved his overall mood and energy levels.

2. Adaptive Cardio Options

Adaptive cardio options, such as recumbent bikes or seated step machines, can be fantastic alternatives for seniors with mobility challenges. These machines provide a way to engage in cardiovascular exercise while seated, reducing the risk of falls and injuries.

Martha, a 70-year-old with balance issues, invested in a recumbent bike for her home. She enjoyed pedaling while watching her favorite shows, making it easier to stick to her routine. As she became more comfortable, she gradually increased the duration and intensity of her workouts, feeling stronger and more confident each day.

3. Group Classes for Support

Many communities offer specialized fitness classes designed for seniors with limited mobility. These classes often focus on gentle movements that promote cardiovascular health while ensuring safety. Joan found a local adaptive fitness class that emphasized seated exercises. The supportive environment and encouragement from the instructor motivated her to push herself while staying safe.

The sense of community she experienced in the class made her look forward to each session, transforming her perception of exercise into a positive and uplifting experience.

Cardio workouts can benefit everyone, regardless of health conditions or physical limitations. By tailoring approaches for seniors with diabetes, respiratory issues, and limited mobility, we can create inclusive environments that encourage all individuals to embrace the joys of aerobic exercise.

The stories of Samuel, Helen, George, and Joan highlight how determination and adaptation can lead to positive health outcomes. With the right support, guidance, and modifications, seniors can successfully engage in cardio workouts that improve their overall well-being and quality of life.

As we continue our journey, the next chapter will delve into the mental health benefits of cardio exercise, showcasing how staying active can lead to enhanced emotional well-being and resilience in later life. Get ready to discover the profound connections between physical activity and mental health!

CONCLUSION

As we reflect on the journey through "Golden Aerobics," it's clear that the power of regular aerobic exercise is transformative, particularly in our later years. This book has explored various aspects of cardio workouts tailored for seniors, offering practical advice, inspiring stories, and techniques designed to enhance health and well-being. In this concluding section, we will emphasize the importance of consistency and embrace the concept of thriving in our golden years.

The Power of Consistency

Consistency is key to maintaining health and vitality as we age. Engaging in regular aerobic exercise not only strengthens the heart and lungs but also contributes to a sense of purpose and community. The stories of individuals like Samuel, Helen, George, and Joan have illustrated how committing to a routine can lead to meaningful changes in their lives.

1. Building a Sustainable Routine

The first step toward thriving is establishing a workout routine that fits seamlessly into your daily life. Whether it's a morning walk, an afternoon swim, or evening chair exercises, find a time that works best for you and make it a non-negotiable part of your schedule. As you commit to this routine, remember the importance of adaptability. Life may throw unexpected challenges your way, but remaining flexible allows you to adjust your workouts while still prioritizing your health.

Martha's journey is a perfect example of this. By exploring different forms of exercise, she found joy and engagement that kept her motivated. It's essential to keep your workouts interesting, whether through varying activities or incorporating friends and family, making exercise something to look forward to rather than a chore.

2. The Mental and Emotional Benefits

In addition to physical health, regular aerobic activity has profound effects on mental and emotional well-being. Exercise releases endorphins, which elevate mood and promote feelings of happiness. It can serve as a powerful antidote to the stresses of life, enhancing your overall quality of life.

For seniors like Joan, who engaged in community fitness classes, the social connections made during workouts provided an invaluable support system. The friendships and camaraderie formed through shared activities not only boosted motivation but also contributed to a richer, more fulfilling life.

Golden Years, Golden Health

Aging is often accompanied by challenges, but it can also be a time of strength, vitality, and joy. Embracing this phase of life with a positive mindset and an active lifestyle can significantly impact your health and happiness.

1. **Celebrating Progress**

It's important to recognize and celebrate the progress you make, no matter how small. Each step forward—whether it's improving endurance, mastering a new exercise, or simply enjoying the moment—is worth acknowledging. Share these victories with friends and family, and don't hesitate to treat yourself for reaching milestones.

Remember Richard, who transformed his fitness routine into a social event by inviting friends to join him for cycling. Not only did he enjoy physical benefits, but he also fostered relationships that enriched his life. Celebrating progress with others can amplify your motivation and make the journey more enjoyable.

2. **Embracing a Holistic Approach**

Thriving in your golden years also involves a holistic approach to health. Incorporating a balanced diet, staying hydrated, and prioritizing sleep are crucial elements of overall wellness. As you engage in cardio, consider the nutritional choices that will fuel your body and support recovery.

Consider creating a meal plan that complements your exercise routine. Many seniors have found success by incorporating more fruits, vegetables, and whole grains into their diets, enhancing their energy levels and promoting heart health.

Appendices

Sample Weekly Cardio Workout Plan for Beginners

- Monday: 30-minute brisk walk

- Tuesday: 20 minutes of chair exercises (upper and lower body)

- Wednesday: 30 minutes of water aerobics or swimming

- Thursday: 20 minutes of cycling (stationary or outdoor)

- Friday: 30 minutes of group dance class

- Saturday: 20 minutes of Tai Chi

- Sunday: Rest or gentle stretching

Recommended Resources

- Fitness Apps: SilverSneakers, MyFitnessPal, Fitbit

- DVDs: "Water Aerobics for Seniors," "Chair Yoga," "Gentle Cardio for Older Adults"

- Websites: Go4Life, AARP Fitness, Senior Fitness

Health Checklists

Symptoms to Watch For During Cardio Workouts:

- Shortness of breath that doesn't improve with rest

- Chest pain or discomfort

- Dizziness or lightheadedness

- Severe fatigue or weakness

When to Seek Medical Advice:

- If you experience persistent symptoms

- After any significant changes in your health status

- Before starting a new exercise program, especially with pre-existing conditions

Final Thoughts

As you embrace the golden years of your life, remember that every step counts. Regular aerobic exercise can profoundly influence your physical and mental health, helping you thrive with strength, vitality, and joy. By committing to a consistent routine, celebrating your progress, and adopting a holistic approach to health, you can navigate the aging process with confidence and enthusiasm.

This book serves as a comprehensive guide, addressing common concerns while providing practical tips to help you engage in cardio workouts safely and effectively. Your journey toward better health starts now—let the rhythms of aerobic exercise carry you into a vibrant future filled with possibilities.